GW01157935

First published in Great Britain in 1996 by
Brockhampton Press,
20 Bloomsbury Street,
London WC1B 3QA.
A member of the Hodder Headline Group.

This series of little gift books was made by Frances Banfield, Andrea P. A. Belloli, Polly Boyd, Kate Brown, Stefano Carantini, Laurel Clark, Penny Clarke, Clive Collins, Jack Cooper, Melanie Cumming, Nick Diggory, John Dunne, Deborah Gill, David Goodman, Paul Gregory, Douglas Hall, Lucinda Hawksley, Maureen Hill, Dicky Howett, Dennis Hovell, Nick Hutchison, Douglas Ingram, Helen Johnson, C.M. Lee, Simon London, Irene Lyford, John Maxwell, Patrick McCreeth, Morse Modaberi, Tara Neill, Sonya Newland, Anne Newman, Grant Oliver, Ian Powling, Terry Price, Michelle Rogers, Mike Seabrook, Nigel Soper, Karen Sullivan and Nick Wells.

ISBN 1 86019 4532

A copy of the CIP data is available from the
British Library upon request.

Produced for Brockhampton Press by Flame Tree Publishing,
a part of The Foundry Creative Media Company Limited,
The Long House, Antrobus Road, Chiswick W4 5HY.

Printed and bound in Italy by L.E.G.O. Spa.

The Funny Book of

SEX

Selected by
Karen Sullivan

Cartoons by

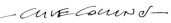

BROCKHAMPTON PRESS

There is more to marriage than
four bare legs in a bed.

Proverb

The difference between sex for money and sex for
free is that sex for money usually costs a lot less.

Brendan Francis

What men call gallantry, and gods adultery,
Is much more common when the climate's sultry.

Lord Byron

Men who never get carried away should be.

Malcolm Forbes

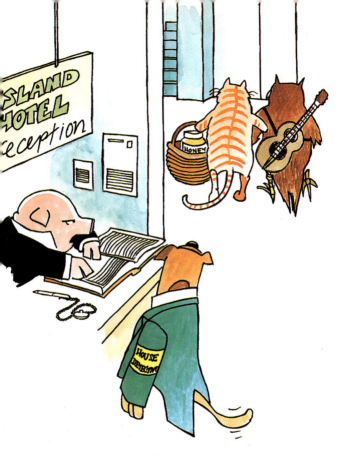

"Keep an eye on those two – they've booked into the
Honeymoon Suite as 'Mr & Mrs Smith'..."

Sex is good, but not as good as fresh sweetcorn.

Garrison Keillor

I love my neighbour as myself, and to avoid coveting my neighbour's wife I desire to be coveted by her — which you know is another thing.

William Congreve

Ever since the young men have owned motorcycles, incest has been dying out.

Max Frisch

Familiarity breeds attempt.

Goodman Ace

Sex is the most fun you can have without smiling.

Anonymous

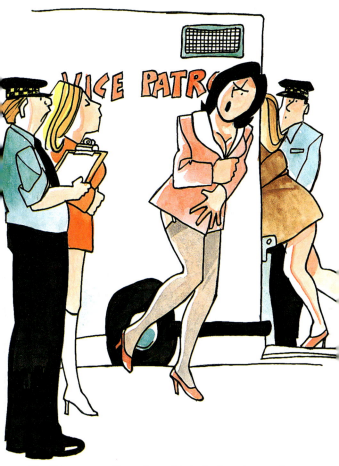

"In fifteen years of marriage, this is the first time you've
shown the slightest interest in my career!"

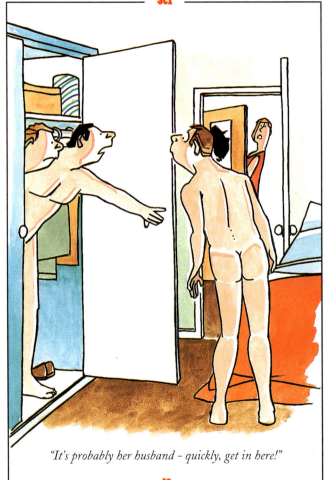

"It's probably her husband – quickly, get in here!"

When I'm good I'm very, very good:
but when I'm bad I'm better.

Mae West

For that same sweet sin of lechery, I would say
as the Friar said: 'A young man and a young
woman in a green arbour in a May morning
— if God do not forgive it, I would.'

Sir John Harrington, **Epigrams**

To live is like to love — all reason is against it,
and all healthy instinct for it.

Samuel Butler, **Notebooks**

Sex is the biggest nothing of all time.

Andy Warhol

For wives, albeit very holy things,
Are bound to suffer patiently at night
Such necessary pleasures as Kings',
Or others who have wedded them with rings.
Her holiness — well she must do without it
Just for a little.

Geoffrey Chaucer, **The Man of Law's Tale**

Contraceptives should be used on
every conceivable occasion.

Spike Milligan

When Pontius wished an edict might be passed
That cuckolds should into the sea be cast,
His wife, assenting, thus replied to him:
'But first, my dear, I'd have you learn to swim.'

Matthew Prior

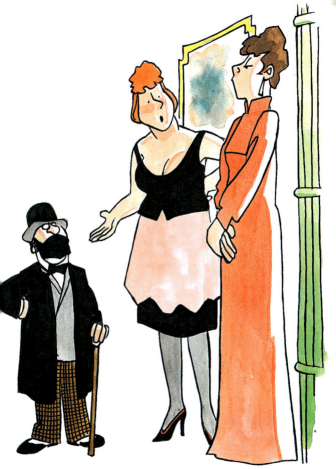

"It's Monsieur Lautrec, Madame –
he insists on only paying half-price..."

13

Charles II does not seem to have
practised birth control. In all he was to
sire thirteen illegitimate children.

Anonymous

Continental people have a sex life;
the English have hot-water bottles.

George Mikes, **How to be an Alien**

A little still she strove, and much repented,
And whispering, 'I will ne'er consent' — consented.

Lord Byron

Last time I tried to make love to my wife
nothing was happening, so I said to her, 'What's
the matter, you can't think of anybody either?'

Rodney Dangerfield

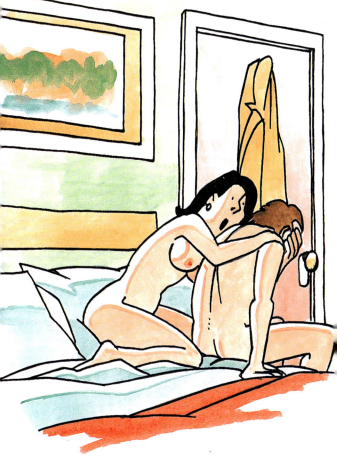

"*What was that? Oh – you suffer from premature ejaculation! Sorry, I couldn't make out what you said – you spoke so fast…*"

She is chaste who was never asked the question.

William Congreve

Middle-aged drunk at party: 'You know,
I'd really like to screw you.'
Diana Dors (surveying him coldly and
wagging an admonishing finger):
'Well, if you do, and I ever find out about it . . .'

Many a promising marriage has foundered in
that cold, forbidding gulf between twin beds.

John Marshall

Don't knock masturbation.
It's sex with someone you love.

Woody Allen

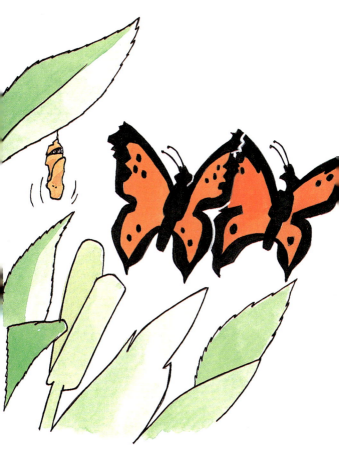

"...and talk about irritable! Mind you, I was just the same when I went through the change..."

Love is the answer, but while you're waiting for the answer, sex raises some pretty good questions.

Woody Allen

Outside every thin woman
is a fat man trying to get in.

Katharine Whitehorn

Marriage is popular because it combines
the maximum of temptation with the
maximum of opportunity.

George Bernard Shaw

Men rarely make passes
At girls wearing glasses.

Dorothy Parker

Women who miscalculate are called 'mothers'.

Abigail van Buren

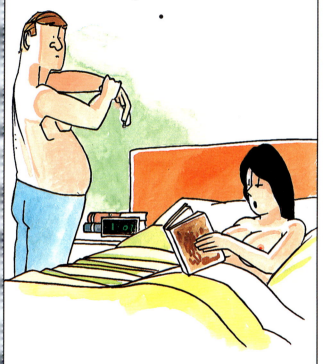

"Well, we certainly know who put the 'pot'
into 'sexpot', don't we?"

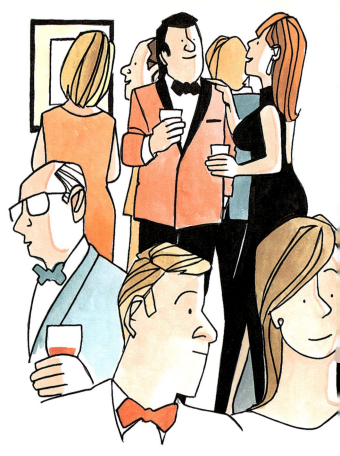

"I'm afraid I'm not much of a conversationalist –
let's go and find the bedroom."

Bette Davis, on a passing starlet well known for
her assiduous cultivation of the casting couch:
'There goes a good time that was had by all.'

Dead birds don't fall out of nests.
*Sir Winston Churchill, when someone told
him his fly was open*

A bird in the bed is worth two in the bushes.
Lambert Jeffries

And down he stooped; upon his back she stood,
Catching a branch, and with a spring she thence
— Ladies, I beg you not to take offence,
I can't embellish, I'm a simple man —
Went up into the tree, and Damian
Pulled up her smock at once and in he thrust.
Geoffrey Chaucer, **The Merchant's Tale**

Culpeper, in the seventeenth century, maintained that the roots of asparagus saturis, boiled in wine, 'stirreth up bodily lust in man or woman.'

A pleasant-looking young cowman was anxious to have his wicked way with the buxom milkmaid. Getting nowhere, he took her one day to watch one of the cows being serviced by the bull, in the hope that the sight would arose thoughts of similar activity in her. 'By Gor,' he said as the bull did his duty, 'I'd love to do just what he's doing now.' 'Why don't you then?' she said with an indifferent shrug. 'It's your cow.'

Kissing is a means of getting two people so close together that they can't see anything wrong with the other.
Rene Yasenek

A terrible thing happened again last night —
nothing.

Phyllis Diller

Commentating on a match involving the player
Renee Richards, who had been a man and had a
sex change operation, Dan Maskell said, in all
innocence, 'Will Miss Richards be serving
with new balls after the changeover, Virginia?'

I'd rather be black than gay: at least if you're black
you don't have to find a way to tell your mother.

American gay activist

Chastity is the most unnatural
of the sexual perversions.

Remy de Gourmont

Is sex dirty? Only if it's done right.
*Woody Allen, **All You've Ever Wanted to Know About Sex***

The radical Northern Irish MP, Bernadette Devlin, as she then was, refused to name the father of her expected child, upon which one of the more acidulous right-wing political commentators observed that, if identified, the man should be charged with having an offensive person on his weapon.

The greatest insult: 'Is it in?'

In the rain at a race meeting, Lester Piggott, seeing a trainer he disliked go past wearing an ankle-length transparent plastic mac, said, 'Ha! 'Tisn't often you see a c*** in a condom, is it?'

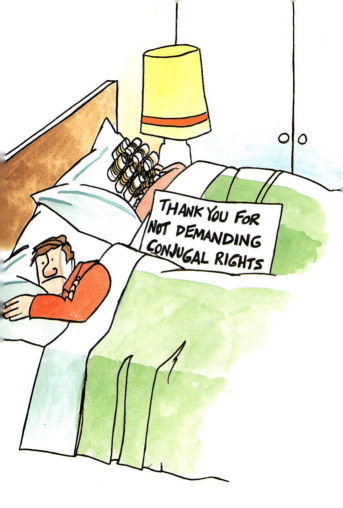

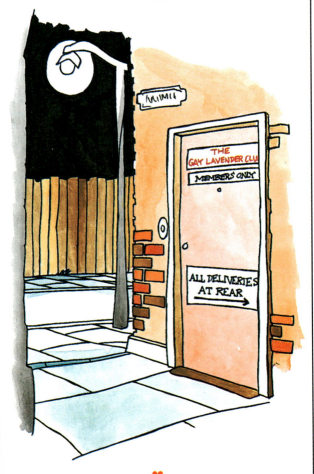

Prostitution gives her an opportunity to meet people. It provides fresh air and wholesome exercise, and it keeps her out of trouble.

Joseph Heller, **Catch 22**

I used to be a virgin, but I gave it up because there was no money in it.

Marsha Warfield

Sweetly innocent newly-wed bride to husband, in bridal suite: 'Now we're married and alone at last, tell me, what is a penis?'
Husband, glad of such a fine opening, removes his trousers and exhibits his own.
Bride, plainly greatly disappointed:
'Christ. All that build-up from the girls, and it's only a prick, but smaller.'

And here's the happy bounding flea —
You cannot tell the he from she.
But she can tell and so can he.

It's better to copulate than never.
Robert Heinlein

It was not the apple on the tree,
but the pair on the ground, I believe,
that caused the trouble in the garden.
M. D. O'Connor

Sex Appeal — Give Generously.
Bumper Sticker

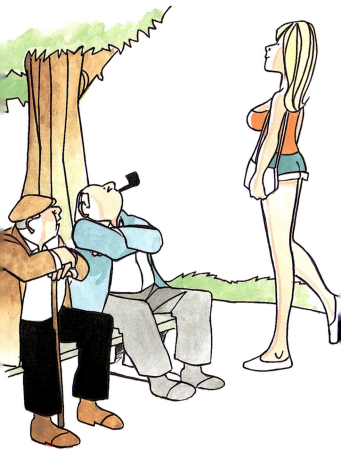

"Oh I remember cold showers,
but I'm damned if I can remember why I took them..."

Sex. In America an obsession.
In other parts of the world a fact.
Marlene Dietrich

Sex is more exciting on the screen and between
the pages than between the sheets.
Andy Warhol

The Englishman can get along with
sex quite perfectly so long as he can
pretend that it isn't sex but something else.
James Agate

Sex is one of the nine reasons for reincarnation.
The other eight are unimportant.
Henry Miller

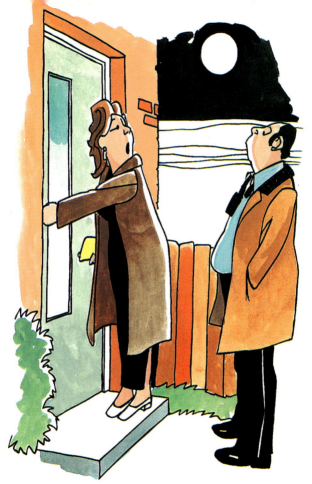

"Bed? Is that some sort of after–dinner joke?"

Don't spend all your energy on sex and all your
money on women; they have destroyed kings.

Proverb

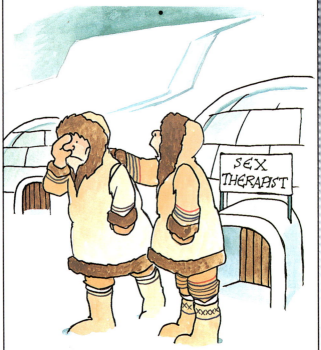

*"Now go home and stop worrying about these old wives' tales –
I assure you, size isn't important..."*

Sex is like money; only too much is enough.

John Updike

Of all sexual aberrations, chastity is the strangest.

Anatole France

He was one of those men who come in a door and make any women with them look guilty.

F. Scott Fitzgerald

Bellhop, bringing a bottle of Scotch and a pack of cigarettes to sweat-bathed and exhausted man in hotel bridal suite: 'Anything else I can get you?'

Man: 'No, thanks.'

Bellhop: 'Anything for the wife?'

Man, after a moment's thought:

'Yes. A postcard and a first-class stamp.'

When grown-ups do it it's kinda dirty.
That's because there's no-one to punish them.

Tuesday Weld

Before we make love, my husband
takes a pain-killer.

Joan Rivers

If it weren't for pickpockets I'd have no sex life at all.

Rodney Dangerfield

Aristocratic young woman brings her
horse back to its stable. The animal is
lathered with sweat and exhausted.
Groom: 'Christ, he's done to the wide.'
Young lady: 'So would you be if you'd been
between my legs for as long as he's been.'

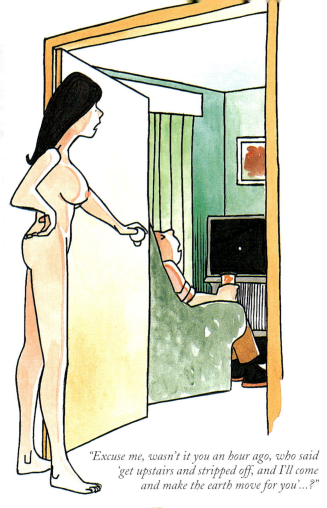

"Excuse me, wasn't it you an hour ago, who said 'get upstairs and stripped off, and I'll come and make the earth move for you'...?"

35

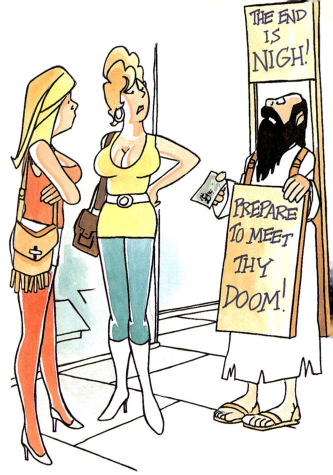

"I want to go out with a bang, not a whimper."

He in a few minutes ravished this fair creature,
or at least would have ravished her, if she had
not, by a timely compliance, prevented him.
Henry Fielding, **Jonathan Wild**

Sex is a misdemeanour.
The less you have, de meaner you get.
Charles Pierce

'I was with a young lady in a taxi, and
I found myself feeling something under
her skirt. It reminded me of Western
Australia. It was triangular, and bushy!'
Barry Humphries,
as Sir Les Patterson, Australian Cultural Attaché

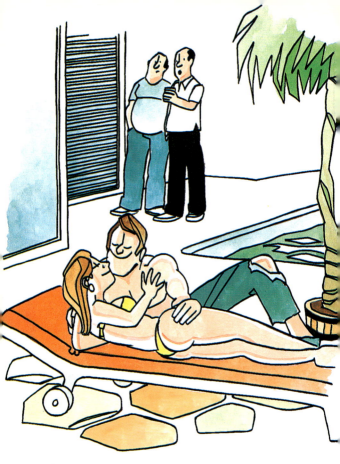

"I hired a handyman to take care of one or two jobs around the house, then one job led to another..."

George Bernard Shaw was sitting at dinner beside a very attractive woman. Shaw asked her, 'Madam, would you go to bed with me for £5000?'

The woman looked astonished and hemmed and hawed a bit.

Shaw then asked, 'Well, how about for £50,000?'

The woman still could not answer.

'Well look,' said Shaw, 'would you go to bed with me for £12?'

'Mr Shaw!' the woman exclaimed.

'What do you think I am?'

Shaw replied, 'We have already established that, Madam. We are just negotiating the price.'

A Treasury of Humour

If sex is such a natural phenomenon, how come there are so many books on how to do it?

Bette Midler

I have so little sex appeal that my
gynaecologist calls me 'Sir'.

Joan Rivers

An eighth-grade boy . . . chose to write a short
paper on the subject of masturbation. His final
paragraph read: 'I don't really see what's wrong
with masturbation. It's always available. It
doesn't cost anything. You don't get anybody
pregnant. You don't catch any diseases. And
you meet a better class of people.'

A Treasury of Humour

It's easy to make a friend.
What's hard is to make a stranger.

Anonymous

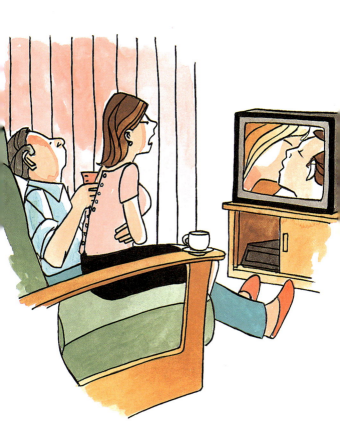

"Forget it, Harry –
the film may be 20 years old, but you're not."

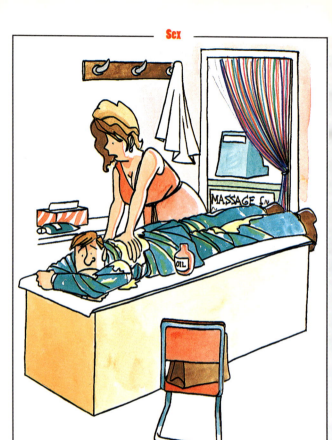

"I'm sorry it's uncomfortable, love – it's just a precaution in case we get raided by the police..."

It must be admitted that we English have sex on the brain, which is a very unfortunate place to have it.

Malcolm Muggeridge

How can a bishop marry?
How can he flirt? The most he can say is,
'I will see you in the vestry after service.'

Sydney Smith

I think making love is the best form of exercise.

Cary Grant

'I've been to bed with well over a hundred women.'
Rosenberg had made some notes of the answers
to all his questions until this last one, at which to
Jake's distinct annoyance he merely nodded.

*Kingsley Amis, **Jake's Thing***

You're the burning heat of a bridal suite in use.
You're the breasts of Venus,
You're King Kong's penis,
You're self-abuse.
You're an arch
In the Rome collection,
You're the starch
In a groom's erection.
Parody of Cole Porter's You're the Top,
believed to be by Porter himself

The reason people sweat is so they
won't catch fire when making love.
Don Rose

He said it was artificial respiration,
but now I find I am to have his child.
Anthony Burgess, **Inside Mr Enderby**

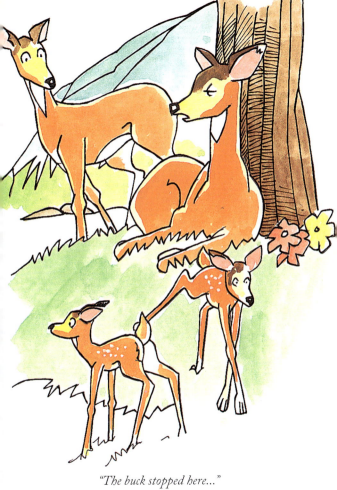

"The buck stopped here..."

On a sofa upholstered in panther skin
Mona did researches in original sin.
William Plomer, **Mews Flat Mona**

Sexual intercourse is the lazy man's
way of masturbating.
Anonymous

The trouble with a virgin is
She's always on the verge.
A virgin is the worst
Her method is reversed
She'll lead a horse to water
And then let him die of thirst.
E. Y. Harburg, **Never Trust a Virgin**

Sex is the gateway to life.
Frank Harris

I am against group sex because I wouldn't
know where to put my elbows.

Martin Cruz Smith

I believe in sex and death — two experiences
that come once in a lifetime.

Woody Allen

Young man at bus-stop seeking to engage young
lady in conversation, decides to open it with the
weather (it's a fresh, breezy day): 'Airy, isn't it?'
Young lady: 'Wot the 'ell did you hexpect?
Hostrich fevvers?'

He took up the pillion
Of his bouncing maid Jillian
And sous'd her like a baggage.

Thomas Triplet, **Ballad**

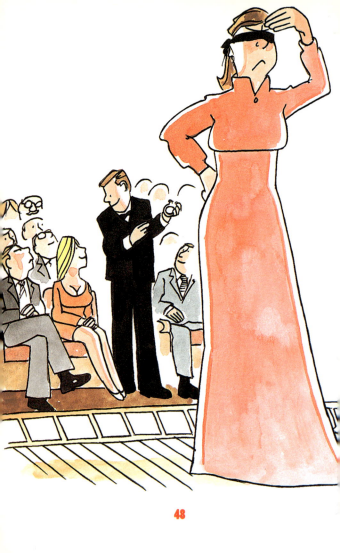

This lad was known as Nicholas the Gallant,
And making love in secret was his talent,
For he was very close and sly, and took
Advantage of his meek and girlish looks.
When things were settled as they thought fit,
And Nicholas had stroked her loins a bit
And kissed her sweetly, he took down his harp
And played away, a merry tune and sharp.
And so the carpenter's wife was truly poked
As if his jealousy to justify.

Geoffrey Chaucer, **The Miller's Tale**

What do you call an uncircumcised Jewish baby?
A girl

Ford decided to manufacture a new,
ultra-cheap model, to be called the Ford Pubic.
It was to be made entirely from old Corsairs.

Your idea of fidelity is not having more
than one man in bed at the same time.
Frederic Raphael, **Darling**

Young man, interrupted in media res in the back
seat of car in a dark street by patrolling policeman.
PC: 'And what do you think you're doing?'
Young man: 'Just necking, officer.'
PC: 'Well just you put your neck back in
your trousers and clear off.'

When self-indulgence has reduced a man to
the shape of Lord Hailsham, sexual continence
requires no more than a sense of the ridiculous.
Reginald Paget, MP, **speech to the House of Commons**

Sex is an emotion in motion.
Mae West

A fast word about oral contraception. I asked a
girl to go to bed with me and she said, 'No'.

Woody Allen

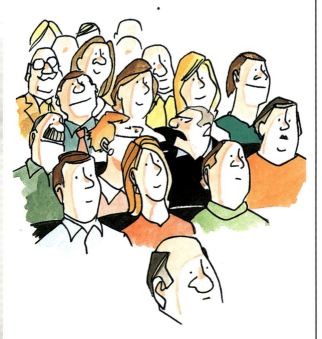

*"I'm warning you, lady – you shove your knee under
my hand just once more..."*

Girl in cinema to boyfriend:
'The man next to me is pulling his wire.'
Boyfriend: 'Take no notice. Just ignore him.'
Girl: 'How can I? He's using my hand.'

A young keep-fit fanatic was doing a hundred push-ups on the beach when a drunk came staggering along, saw him, watched bemused for a while, then collapsed in a paroxysm of laughter. The athlete glared round and snapped, 'What the hell are you laughing at?' When the drunk had finally managed to suppress his laughter he spluttered, 'Don't look now, shonny, but shomeone's shtolen your girl.'

It serves me right for putting all
my eggs in one bastard.
Dorothy Parker, **on her abortion**

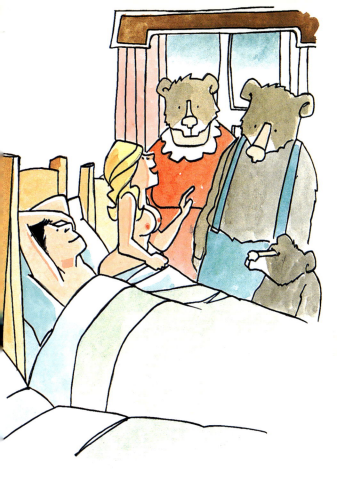

"...but the bed is just right!"

Lechery, sir [drink] provokes and
unprovokes: it provokes the desire
but it takes away the performance.
William Shakespeare, **Macbeth**

Masturbation is the thinking man's television.
Christopher Hampton, **The Philanthropist**

I've been around so long I knew
Doris Day before she was a virgin.
Groucho Marx

Son: Lesbianism?
Well, I come across it in literature.
Mother: Well, I hope it is in
literature and not in Halifax.
Alan Bennett, **Me! I'm Afraid of Virginia Woolf**

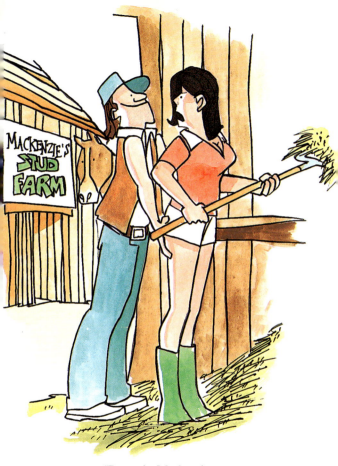

"Dammit, Mackenzie –
can't you ever think of anything but work?"

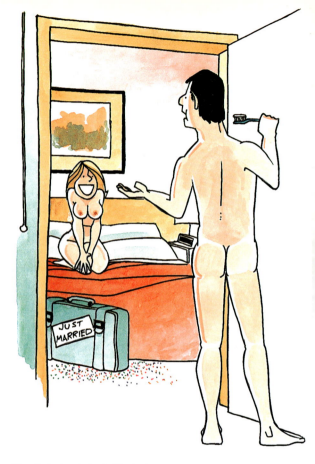

"Look, losing it isn't like losing a tooth – there'll be no money under the pillow in the morning..."

Three daughters were all married on the same day. That night their parents listened at their bedroom doors, and heard the first daughter laughing, the second crying and the third silent.

In the morning the mother took them aside one by one and asked them to explain.

'Well,' said the first, 'you always told me to laugh if something tickled me.'

'Well,' said the second, 'you always said there was no shame in crying if something hurt me.'

'Well,' said the third, 'you always said it was rude to talk with my mouth full.'

Man pouring drink: 'Say when.'
Woman: 'After this drink.'

At certain times I like sex — like after a cigarette.
Rodney Dangerfield

The act of sex, gratifying as it may be,
is God's joke on humanity.

Bette Davis

As a test of your relationship with the world, sex
could never be a patch on being murdered. That's
when someone really does risk his life for you.

Quentin Crisp, **How to Become a Virgin**

There are a number of mechanical devices
which increase sexual arousal, especially amongst
women. Chief among these is the Mercedes
Benz 380SL convertible.

P. J. O'Rourke, **Modern Manners**

If all the girls attending it were laid end to end,
I wouldn't be at all surprised.

Dorothy Parker, **on the Yale Prom**

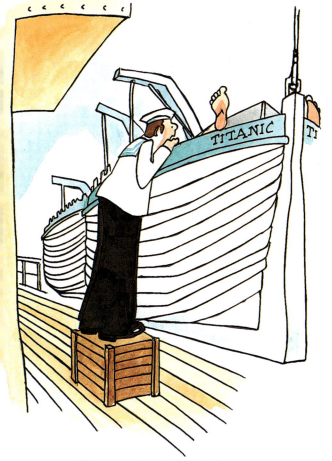

*"You two can't make love in there –
suppose we had an emergency..."*

My father told me all about the birds and the bees.
The liar — I went steady with a woodpecker
till I was twenty-one.

Bob Hope

Now let us sport us while we may,
And now, like amorous birds of prey,
Let us roll all our strength and all
Our sweetness up into one ball,
And tear our pleasures with rough strife
Thorough the iron gates of life.

Andrew Marvell, **To His Coy Mistress**

Sex will outlive us all.

Sam Goldwyn

Acknowledgements:

The Publishers wish to thank everyone who gave permission to reproduce the quotes in this book. Every effort has been made to contact the copyright holders, but in the event that an oversight has occurred, the publishers would be delighted to rectify any omissions in future editions of this book.*A Treasury of Humor*, by Eric W. Johnson, published by Ivy Book, Ballantine Books © Eric W. Johnson, 1989; George Bernard Shaw, reprinted courtesy of the Society of Authors on behalf of the Estate of George Bernard Shaw; J. D. Salinger, reprinted courtesy of Penguin Books; *Good News Study Bible*, published by Thomas Nelson, 1986, extracts reprinted with their kind permission; *Penguin Book of Japanese Verse*, translated by Geoffrey Bownas and Anthony Thwaite, published by Penguin 1964, and reprinted with their permission; Garrison Keillor, reprinted courtesy of Faber & Faber and Viking Penguin; Dorothy Parker quotes from *The Best of Dorothy Parker*, first published by Methuen in 1952, reprinted by Gerald Duckworth & Co., © Dorothy Parker, 1956, 1957, 1958, 1959, renewed; Quotations attributed to Mike Seabrook were supplied by Mr Seabrook and printed with his permission; P. G. Wodehouse extracts © P. G. Wodehouse, reprinted courtesy of Herbert Jenkins and Penguin Books; Joan Rivers and others quoted in *1911 Best Things Anybody Ever Said*, by Robert Byrne, published by Ballantine Books © 1988 Robert Byrne, reprinted by permission of Random House, Inc., New York, and Random House of Canada Limited, Toronto.

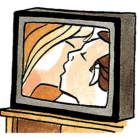